easy
pilates

any age • any place • any time

Mina Stephens

Consultant Osteopath
Sean Durkan

Illustrated by
Juliet Percival

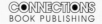

CONNECTIONS
BOOK PUBLISHING

A CONNECTIONS EDITION
This edition published in Great Britain in 2008 by
Connections Book Publishing Limited
St Chad's House, 148 King's Cross Road
London WC1X 9DH
www.connections-publishing.com

British Library Cataloguing-in-Publication data available on request.

ISBN 978-1-85906-268-5

1   3   5   7   9   10   8   6   4   2

Phototypeset in Meta using QuarkXPress on Apple Macintosh
Printed in China

Contents

Introduction

In the early twentieth century, Joseph Pilates developed an innovative fitness system based on a number of forms of exercise from both the Eastern and Western worlds. This method, known today as 'Pilates', set a precedent that has had great influence on our modern-day idea of mind–body fitness.

I have been practising Pilates for more than twenty years and have seen for myself how this exercise system has been influenced by sports biomechanics and, unfortunately, the passive lifestyles that the majority of us have adopted. However, no matter what variation is offered, the true core principles of Joseph's original teachings remain constant.

This book is written with these new concepts in mind, and so it is a modern interpretation of traditional Pilates. Here, Pilates is presented in its most simplistic form, designed to help inspire you to gain control of your body and well-being using a 'back to basics' approach, making it accessible to all.

Pilates is a safe and effective form of exercise that can be practised at home or at the gym. Regular practice will help you improve your posture and core strength, breathing and circulation, flexibility and coordination – the list goes on. It sounds too good to be true, but, if you commit yourself to a regular routine, it really works!

All you need is an exercise mat and enough room to lie down and stretch out. It also helps to have a small towel handy to use as a support for your head when practising some of the exercises. This fitness programme is not suitable for pregnant women or for those with serious neck or back injuries. Always consult your doctor if you have any questions or health concerns.

How to use this book

The specific sequences are designed so that you can structure your fitness regime around your busy schedule. My advice is that you set aside a fixed time two or three times a week, and stick to it! I find that my private clients who schedule their appointments for the same time every week are the most committed and achieve the fastest results.

Start with the 45-minute session. This will build endurance and body-awareness skills, while providing a well-balanced routine that works and stretches every muscle in your body. Once you've gained confidence, you can move onto the shorter sessions for more specific needs. The 20-minute Wake Up and Go sequence helps you to feel energized and relaxed. If you're experiencing tension in the shoulders, neck or lower back, try one of the simplified 10-minute sessions to strengthen and stretch these problem areas.

To inspire your practice, the book jacket folds out into a wall chart showing the poses in sequence. You can place it wherever you practise Pilates, for easy reference.

It is vital that you focus on your breathing and posture when practising Pilates, to ensure that you benefit fully from the routines and – most importantly – avoid injury. So please read the following information carefully before you attempt any of the exercises.

Deep breathing

Breathing is one of the major principles of Pilates. It is imperative to learn how to breathe properly from the diaphragm (the primary breathing muscle). Breathing high up into the chest and lifting your shoulders on the inhale (using your secondary breathing muscles) causes undue stress in the shoulder and neck muscles. Whatever you're doing, you should breathe so that on the inhale, your lungs fill up with air allowing the stomach to naturally extend outwards. Then, on the exhale, the stomach deflates back towards the spine.

When practising Pilates, breathe in through your nose and out through your mouth. Take a slow, deep breath, low and wide into the lungs, expanding the ribcage out to the sides and back. On the exhale, simultaneously draw up through your pelvic floor (the muscles that help stop the flow of urine) and squeeze your abdominal muscles back towards your spine, as if tightening a belt around your waist. This will activate core muscles, which include the pelvic floor, deep abdominals and deep back muscles (*see opposite*). Understanding the direct link between correct breathing and the activation of these muscles while exercising will actually help you to develop core strength.

Another key factor is the coordination of correct body alignment and pelvic stability. The goal is to stabilize the pelvis and shoulders in a neutral position while exercising, to help avoid the risk of injury. Maintaining the natural curves in your back (known as 'neutral spine') will assist the strengthening of core postural muscles, encouraging the spine and limbs to stretch and lengthen.

Understanding the arrows
The meanings of the arrows used in some of the exercises are as follows:

A solid arrow tells you to move the relevant part of the body in the direction shown.

A dotted arrow tells you to keep the relevant part of the body fixed in a particular position.

The use of key muscles in Pilates

FRONT VIEW

REAR VIEW

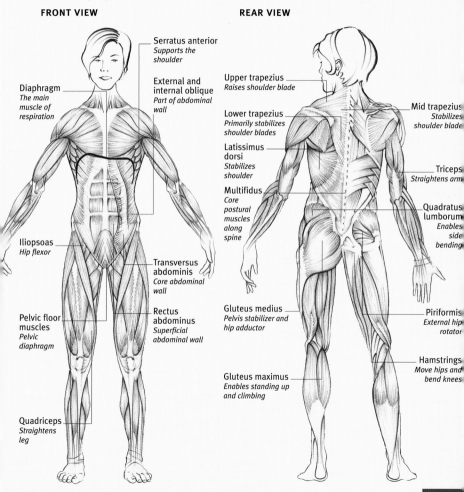

Serratus anterior
Supports the shoulder

External and internal oblique
Part of abdominal wall

Diaphragm
The main muscle of respiration

Iliopsoas
Hip flexor

Transversus abdominis
Core abdominal wall

Rectus abdominus
Superficial abdominal wall

Pelvic floor muscles
Pelvic diaphragm

Quadriceps
Straightens leg

Upper trapezius
Raises shoulder blade

Lower trapezius
Primarily stabilizes shoulder blades

Latissimus dorsi
Stabilizes shoulder

Multifidus
Core postural muscles along spine

Gluteus medius
Pelvis stabilizer and hip adductor

Gluteus maximus
Enables standing up and climbing

Mid trapezius
Stabilizes shoulder blade

Triceps
Straightens arm

Quadratus lumborum
Enables side bending

Piriformis
External hip rotator

Hamstrings
Move hips and bend knees

full-length sequence

45-MINUTE SESSION

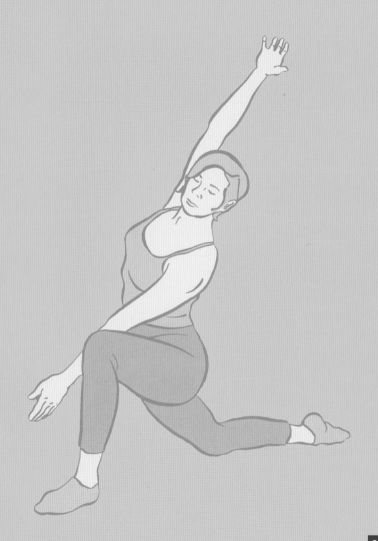

① **Breathwork**

Helps activate deep postural muscles • Focuses on body alignment and neutral spine

Lie on your back with your knees bent, feet hip-width apart and arms relaxed by your sides. Keeping the shoulders relaxed, gently lengthen the back of your neck and your tailbone, sinking them into the mat so that your spine is resting in neutral. You can find your neutral spine position by slipping one hand under your lower back, into the small space between your body and the floor. Don't over-arch the back.

1 Slowly inhale through your nose, drawing the air deep into your lungs and into the sides of the ribcage – think low and wide.

1

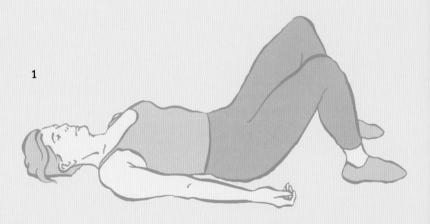

2 Exhale through your mouth and simultaneously pull up through your pelvic floor while squeezing the abdominals down towards your spine as if you are tightening a belt around your waist – try to draw the front of your ribs together at the end of the exhale. Think 'navel to spine' without rocking the pelvis or hunching the shoulders.

Repeat ten times.

Throughout this exercise the breath should not be forced. Create ease and flow, even while engaging the core muscles.

• This breathing technique will be incorporated into the exercise sequences that follow.

2

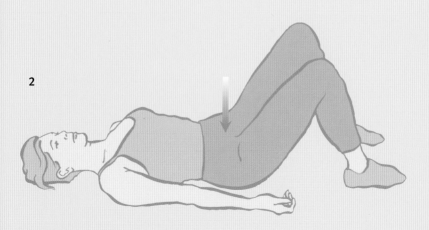

❷ The pelvic rock

Mobilizes the pelvis and lower spine • Coordinates breathwork with movement

The pelvic rock is very similar to the breathwork exercise shown on the previous page, but here the pelvis rocks forwards and backwards slightly.

Lie on your back with your knees bent, feet hip-width apart and arms relaxed by your sides. Relax your shoulders and spine into the neutral position by gently lengthening the back of your neck and your tailbone, sinking them into the mat.

1 Inhale deeply, drawing the breath into the sides of the ribcage.

1

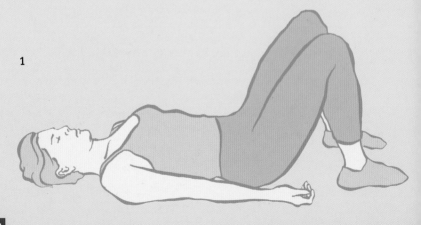

2 As you exhale, draw up through your pelvic floor, engage your
   abdominals (not your buttocks or hip flexors), lowering them towards
   the spine, and tilt the pelvis towards the navel slowly rolling the tailbone
   off the floor. Inhale and release the tailbone back to the neutral position,
   taking care not to over-exaggerate the curve in the lower spine.

Repeat step 2 ten times.

2

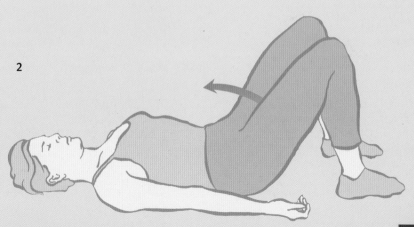

③ The pelvic tilt

Mobilizes and lengthens all the muscles in the spine • Focuses on deep abdominal connection

This is a continuation of the pelvic rock, but now utilizing the whole spine.

Lie on your back in the neutral position with your knees bent, feet hip-width apart and arms relaxed by your sides.

1 Inhale deeply, drawing the breath into the sides of the ribcage.

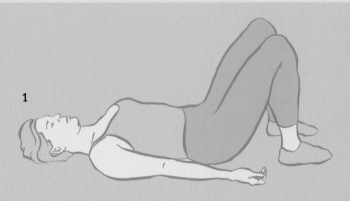

2 With a long, sustained exhale, engage your pelvic floor and abdominals and tilt the pelvis towards the navel – the abdominals initiate this movement, not the buttocks. Slowly peel your back off the mat, rolling up through one vertebra at a time. Take care not to lift your pelvis too high as this will cause the back to over-arch. Keep your shoulders and neck relaxed.

3 Inhale, holding this position. Then, as you slowly exhale, roll down one vertebra at a time, lowering the back to the floor, stretching and lengthening through the spine.

Repeat ten times.

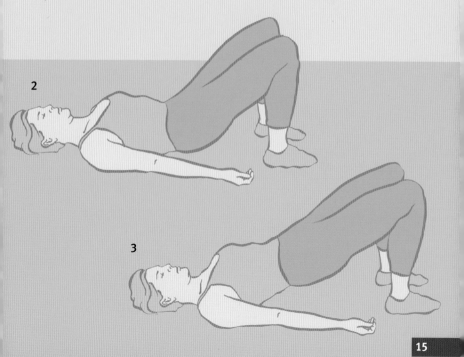

❹ Knee drops

Stabilizes the pelvis • Mobilizes the hip joints

This exercise requires you to stabilize one side of your body, while mobilizing the other.

1 Lie on your back in the neutral position with your knees bent, feet hip-width apart and arms relaxed by your sides. Focus on the pelvic floor and abdominal muscles to maintain a neutral pelvis throughout. Keep your neck relaxed.

2 As you inhale, relax one knee out to the side, making sure the opposite hip doesn't lift from the floor.

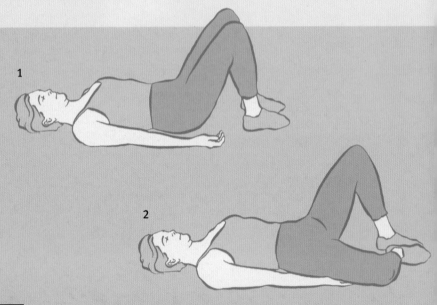

3 Exhale and extend the leg along the mat, taking care not to arch the back – think of the stretch starting from the hip. Keep the leg extended as you inhale.

4 As you exhale, pull the navel down towards the spine, and, primarily using the abdominal muscles, bend the leg back to the starting position keeping the foot on the mat.

Repeat ten times with each leg.

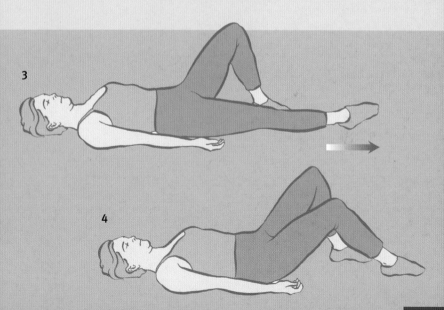

❺ Arm reaches

Mobilizes and stabilizes the shoulder blades • Stretches the muscles in the upper and mid back

Lie on your back in the neutral position with your knees bent, feet hip-width apart. Lengthen the back of the neck by drawing the shoulders down away from the ears. The shoulder blades should feel wide apart and flat against the mat. This is your fixed neutral shoulder position.

1 Inhale and stretch the arms up towards the ceiling, pulling the shoulder blades apart to open the upper back. Take care not to hunch the shoulders up towards the ears.

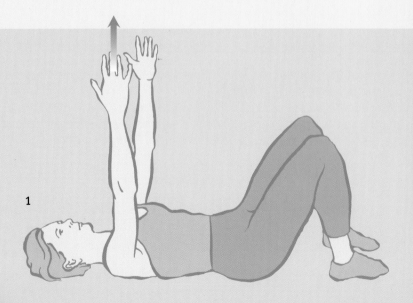

1

2 As you exhale, drop the shoulder blades back to the neutral starting position. Make sure you don't arch the back in response to these subtle movements.

Repeat ten times, concentrating on maintaining the width across the upper back and chest.

2

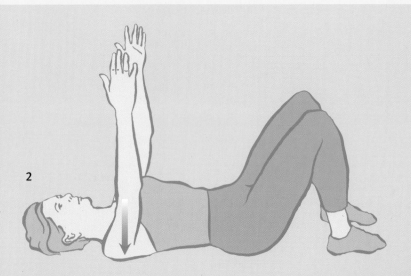

❻ Around the world

Mobilizes the shoulder joints • Opens up the chest and mid back

Caution: Avoid this exercise if you have a history of shoulder dislocation.

For this exercise you may wish to place a small folded towel under your head to keep your neck aligned with the upper back.

1 Lie on your right-hand side with your knees bent, legs together and your arms stretched out in front of you with your palms together.

2 Keeping your knees together, in a slow fluid motion begin to circle the left arm around towards your head. The eyes should follow the arm, but keep your head relaxed and resting on the towel.

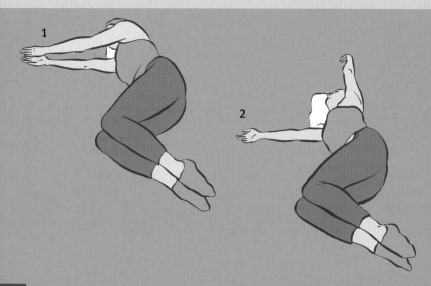

3 Continue to move the arm around, flattening both shoulder blades against the mat as you reach the floor behind you. You should feel a wonderful stretch in the mid back as you gently twist the spine.

4 Finally, bring the arm around past the upper hip and back to the starting position.

Repeat ten times, then complete ten rotations in the opposite direction. Turn over and repeat on the other side.

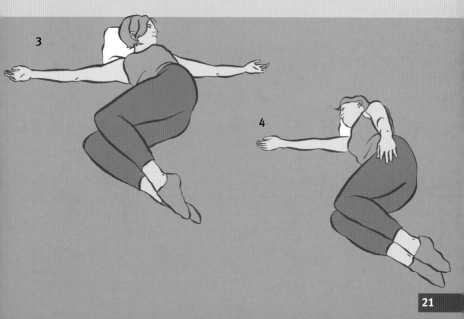

❼ Hip rolls

Strengthens the abdominal muscles • Stabilizes the shoulder blades •
Opens up the chest • Improves spinal flexibility

Lie on your back in the neutral position with your knees bent, legs
pressed together.

1 Reach your arms out to the sides, your shoulders pulling away from
your ears.

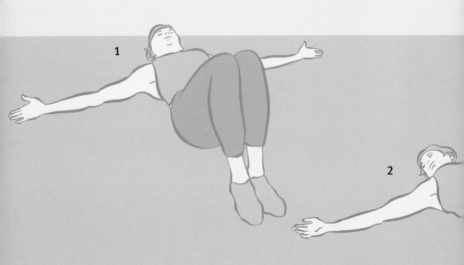

2 As you inhale, roll your knees over to the left-hand side and turn your head to face towards the right, keeping both shoulder blades connected to the mat. Take care not to arch the back.

3 Exhale, engaging your pelvic floor and abdominal muscles, and return the knees and head to the starting position. Repeat to the other side.

Complete the exercise five times.

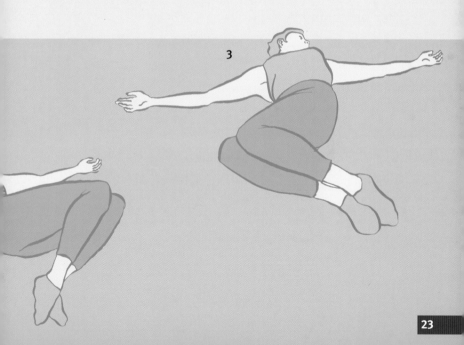

❽ Abdominal preps

Strengthens core abdominal and postural muscles • Stabilizes the neutral spine

Lie on your back in the neutral position with your knees bent, feet hip-width apart. Clasp your hands behind your head with your elbows raised off the mat slightly.

1   Inhale and lengthen the back of your neck by gently nodding the chin towards the chest.

1

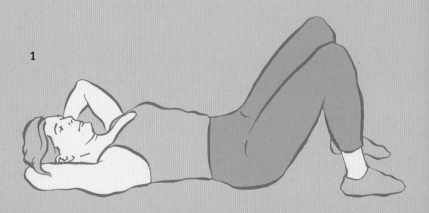

2 As you exhale, draw your shoulders down away from your ears, pull up through your pelvic floor and squeeze your abdominals back towards your spine. Maintaining this fixed position, curl your head and shoulders up off the floor. Inhale, still squeezing your abdominal muscles, then exhale and lower the upper body to the floor. This exercise may take some practice.

Repeat ten times.

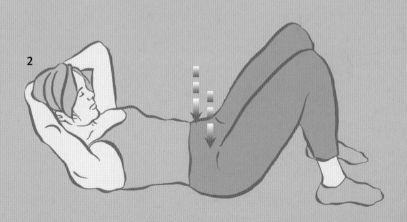

⑨ Hundreds

Promotes breath control • Strengthens abdominal and postural muscles •
Stabilizes shoulders and pelvis

To help release tension in your neck, place a small folded towel underneath your head before you start. Lie on your back in the neutral position with your knees bent, feet hip-width apart.

1   Place your arms by your sides, slightly raised off the mat, palms facing downwards. Start pumping your arms up and down in a continuous movement, as though you're slapping a puddle on the floor. Focus on keeping your breathing constant.

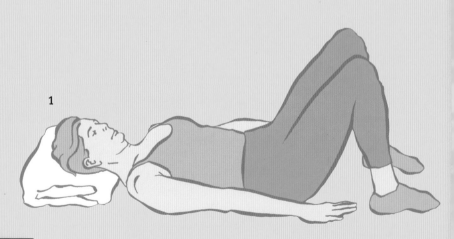

1

2 Inhale deeply for a count of five, then exhale for a count of five, pulling up through your pelvic floor and squeezing your abdominals. Keep your arms strong and stretch your fingers towards your feet. Don't allow the neck to become tense. Each time you exhale, feel all the air being squeezed out of your lungs.

Continue for ten inhales and exhales.

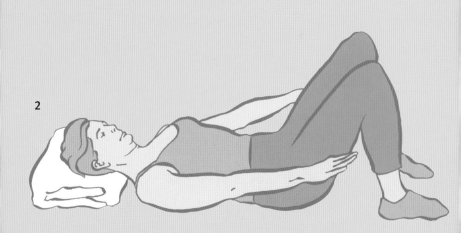

2

⑩ Roll-ups

Mobilizes the spine • Strengthens the abdominals

Sitting with your knees bent and your feet hip-width apart, reach your arms out in front of you level with the shoulders.

1 Focus on lengthening your spine upwards while sliding the shoulder blades down towards the hips. Inhale deeply into the ribcage.

2 Exhale, squeezing your abdominals back towards your spine, and start to roll your torso backwards off the pelvis, leading with your lower spine (not the shoulders). Stop once you are leaning back

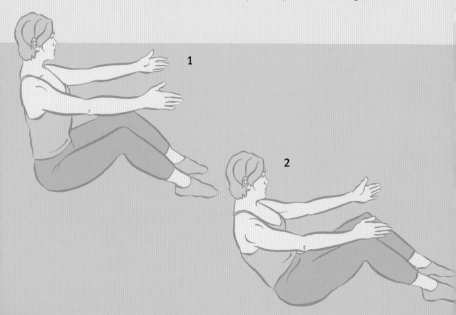

about halfway, your arms held forwards. Don't allow the chest to collapse. Keep your feet imprinted on the mat. Inhale, holding this deep curve in your lower back.

3 As you exhale, connect your pelvic floor and abdominals and slowly roll your body up and over your hips, reaching your hands past your heels. Maintain the contraction of the abdominal muscles.

4 Inhale, elongating the spine to return to the starting position.

Repeat ten times.

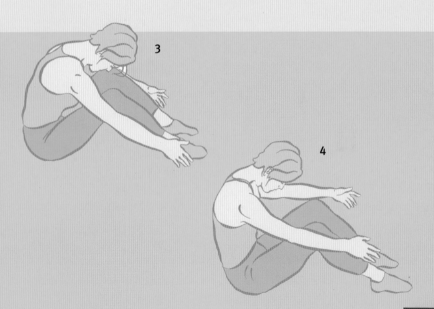

⓫ Single-leg circles

Mobilizes the hip joints • Stretches the hip and thigh muscles •
Strengthens the abdominal muscles

Lie on your back with your arms relaxed by your sides.

1 Extend your left leg up towards the ceiling, keeping it directly over the
   pelvis, and lengthen your right leg straight along the floor. Make sure
   your hips are level. If you find it difficult to straighten your leg, bend
   the knee slightly.

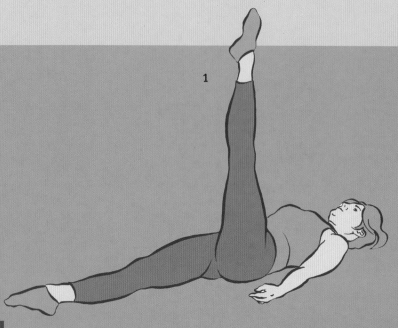

1

2 Now, imagine you are drawing circles – about the size of dinner plates – on the ceiling with your toes, while stirring the leg in the hip socket. Squeeze your abdominals as you circle the leg, making sure the right hip remains fixed to the floor. Try to keep your shoulders and neck relaxed throughout the movement.

Circle the leg five times clockwise then five times anti-clockwise. Repeat with the right leg.

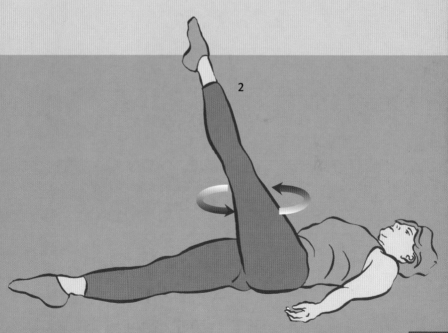

⑫ Rolling like a ball

Maintains abdominal connection while mobilizing the spine

Begin by sitting on the floor at the front of your mat.

1 Draw the knees up towards the chest with your toes resting on the
   mat. Your body weight should be on your tailbone slightly. Try to create
   a deep scoop with your abdominals. Place your hands on the outside
   of the calf muscles.

1

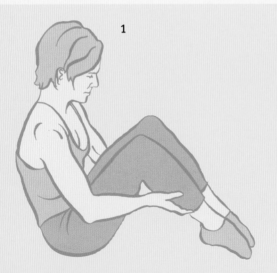

2

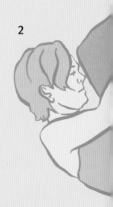

2 Maintaining this scooped position with your chin pointed down towards your chest, inhale and begin to roll back onto your shoulder blades – don't allow your head to touch the mat.

3 Immediately roll back up to the position shown in step 1. As you roll up, exhale using your abdominal muscles. You will find it easier to roll through your spine if you keep your heels close to your buttocks and your chin towards your chest.

Repeat ten times.

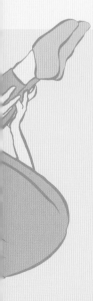

3

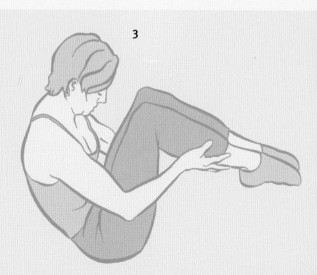

⓭ Single-leg stretches

Strengthens the abdominals • Works and lengthens the leg muscles while stabilizing the shoulders and hips

To help release tension in your neck, place a small folded towel underneath your head before you start. Lie on your back and bend both knees into your chest.

1 Hold onto the left knee with both hands and extend the right leg as shown. Draw the shoulders down, away from the ears, and lift your elbows away from the body slightly. Inhale.

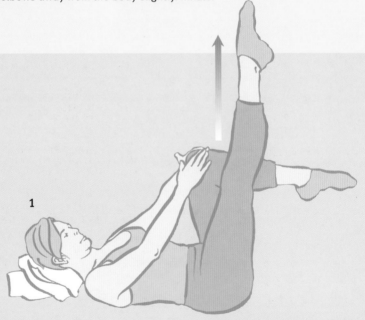

2 As you exhale, switch legs, placing your hands on the right knee and extending the left leg. As you do so, squeeze your abdominal muscles to prevent the pelvis from shifting and the back from arching.

Repeat five times.

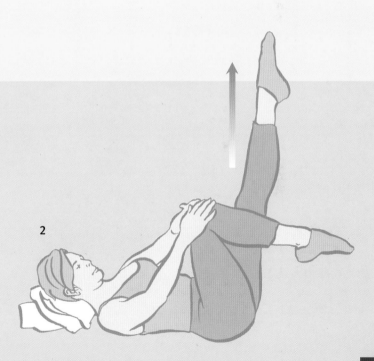

2

⑭ The criss-cross

Strengthens the core abdominal and oblique muscles • Stabilizes the shoulders

Lie on your back with your hands clasped behind your head.

1 Raise your legs so that your knees are directly over your hips. Gently pull your shoulders away from your ears and down towards the hips. Lift the head and shoulders off the mat, keeping the elbows wide. Take care not to arch the back. Inhale to prepare.

2 As you exhale, draw up through your pelvic floor, squeeze your abdominals back towards your spine and extend the left leg at

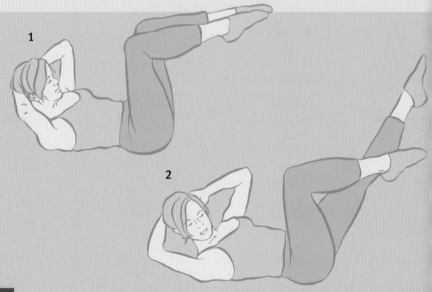

an angle, as shown. At the same time, twist your torso towards the right, maintaining the wide elbow position. As you stretch the leg, keep the pelvis centred. Don't allow the hips to rock.

3 Inhale to bring the extended leg and the torso back to centre.

4 As you exhale, switch sides, focusing on the abdominal connection.

Repeat ten times, alternating sides.

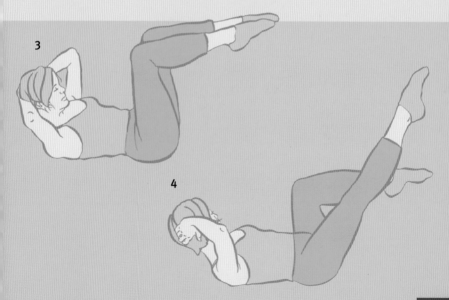

⑮ The spine stretch

Mobilizes and lengthens the spine • Stretches the hamstrings

Begin by sitting with your legs slightly wider than hip-width apart, knees slightly bent.

1   Reach your arms out in front of you, level with your shoulders. Focus on lengthening your spine upwards and draw your shoulders down towards the hips. If you find this difficult, bend your knees a little more, keeping your feet flat on the floor. Inhale deeply into the ribcage.

2   As you exhale, squeeze the abdominals back towards the spine and curve your whole spine forwards, reaching the hands towards the toes

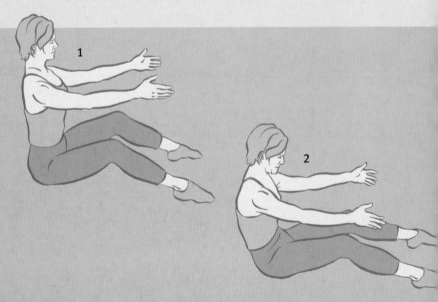

– imagine that your waist is being pulled back as you stretch forwards. Try not to hunch the shoulders – keep them away from the ears.

3 Inhale, keeping the abdominal muscles scooped in, and focus on maximizing the stretch.

4 Exhale and roll the spine back up, one vertebra at a time, to return to the upright position shown in step 1.

Repeat ten times.

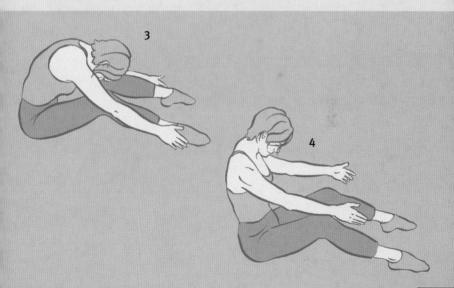

⑯ The saw

Strengthens the oblique muscles • Stabilizes the pelvis • Stretches the upper back muscles

Begin by sitting with your legs slightly wider than hip-width apart, with your knees slightly bent.

1   Reach your arms straight out to the sides and pull your shoulders away from the ears, widening the chest and upper back.

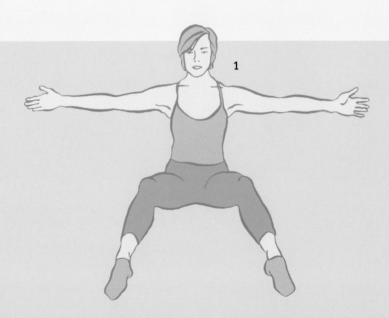

2 Inhale deeply into the ribcage, growing taller through your spine. Now twist the upper body and arms to the right without moving the hips.

3 Exhale and look back towards the right arm as you stretch the left arm down the outside of the right leg, squeezing your navel towards the spine. Feel an oppositional stretch in the arms as you finish the exhale. Inhale to return to the upright position shown in step 1, lengthening your waist.

Repeat ten times, alternating sides.

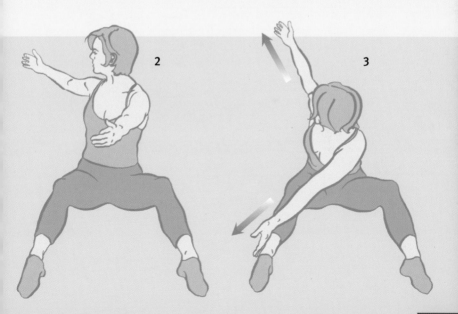

⑰ Leg lifts

Works the body unilaterally while stabilizing the shoulders • Strengthens the back, abdominals and leg muscles

Lie on your right-hand side with your legs stretched out in line with your hips and shoulders.

1 Support your head with your right hand, resting your elbow on the mat, and press the left hand down firmly in front of your ribcage. Lengthen the neck by pressing the left shoulder down towards your hips. It is important to maintain this shoulder stability throughout the exercise as this will help you to balance. Inhale and lengthen both legs away from your hips.

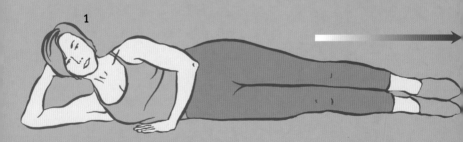

2 As you exhale, squeeze the navel back towards the spine and lift both legs off the mat, pressing the backs of your inner thighs together tightly and stretching out through your toes. Inhale and focus on controlling your whole body as you lower your legs to the mat.

Complete the exercise ten times, then repeat on the other side.

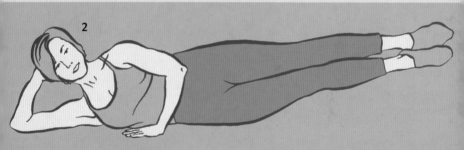

⑱ Superman

Stabilizes the shoulder blades • Strengthens the core abdominal and back muscles • Works the hamstrings and buttocks

On all fours, position your hands directly underneath your shoulders and place your knees in line with your hips.

1   Look down towards the floor so that your head is in line with the neck and draw the shoulders away from the ears. Lengthen your spine in both directions. Inhale deeply into the ribcage.

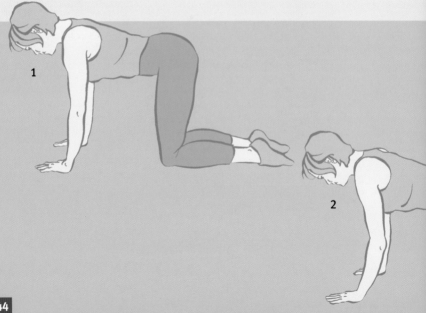

2 As you exhale, pull up through your pelvic floor and squeeze your abdominals back towards your spine. Then lift your right leg off the floor, extending it straight back in line with the hip. Try not to shift your weight to the left or lift the right hip – it's important to maintain the neutral pelvis. Inhale, holding this position.

3 Exhale and raise the left hand. Once again, concentrate on keeping your weight centred and your shoulders pressed down, away from your ears. As you inhale, return your arm and leg to the starting position shown in step 1.

Repeat ten times, alternating sides.

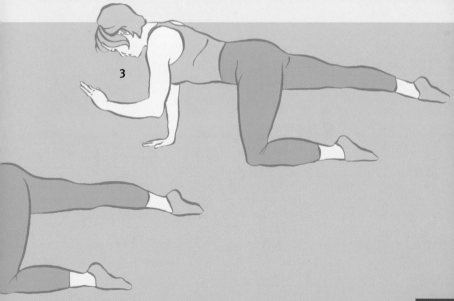

⑲ The cobra

Strengthens the core abdominal and back muscles • Stabilizes the shoulder blades

Begin by lying face down with your legs hip-width apart.

1 Place your palms face down next to your shoulders and rest your elbows by your sides, close to the ribs. Gently press the elbows down into the mat. Slide the shoulder blades downwards and outwards towards your hips, fixing the shoulders away from the ears. Look down to lengthen the back of the neck, and stretch the spine in both directions. Inhale, focusing on this spinal stretch.

1

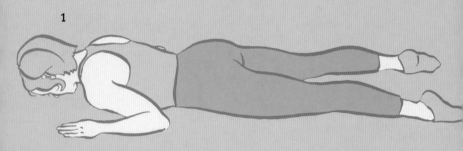

2 As you exhale, pull up through your pelvic floor and squeeze your navel towards the spine. Lift the chest off the mat and keep your elbows pressed down. It is imperative to maintain the connection in the abdominals at this point to ensure sufficient support for the lower back. Inhale and lower the body back down to the mat.

Repeat ten times.

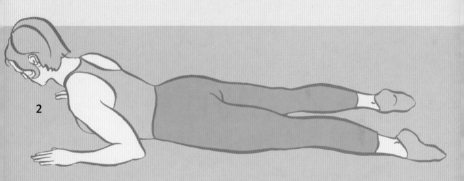

2

⑳ The star

Strengthens the core muscle groups • Lengthens the spine • Works the hamstrings and buttocks

Begin by lying face down on the mat.

1 Place your legs hip-width apart and extend your arms out in front of you, shoulder-width apart, palms flat on the mat. Look down to lengthen the back of the neck and pull your shoulders down away from the ears. Inhale, fixing the shoulder blades down towards the hips.

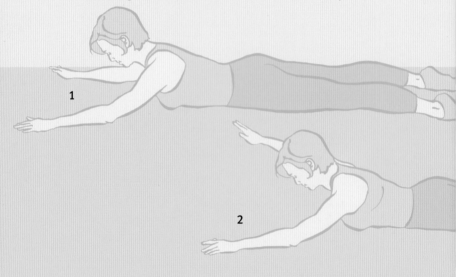

2 As you exhale, pull up through the pelvic floor and squeeze the navel back towards the spine. This will ensure that the lower back is adequately supported. Simultaneously, lift and lengthen the right arm and left leg. Make sure both hips remain on the mat. Inhale and lower the arm and leg back down to the mat.

3 Repeat step 2 with the left arm and right leg.

Repeat five times.

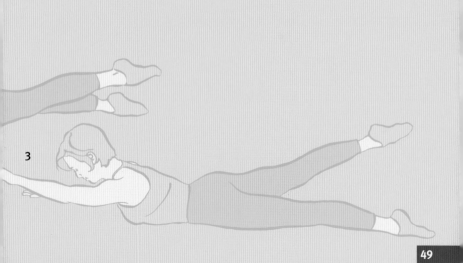

3

㉑ The cat

Mobilizes and stretches the spine • Stabilizes the shoulders

On all fours, position your hands directly underneath the shoulders and place your knees in line with the hips.

1 Look down towards the floor so that your head is in line with the neck and draw the shoulders away from the ears. Lengthen your spine in both directions. Inhale deeply into the ribcage.

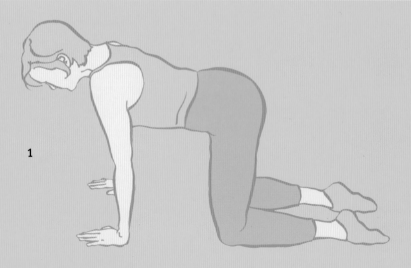

1

2 Exhale, pulling up through your pelvic floor, and squeeze your abdominals back towards your spine, lifting the spine up towards the ceiling. At the top of this lift, inhale, gently pressing the hands down into the mat to achieve a greater stretch. Exhale and relax the spine down to the starting position.

Repeat ten times.

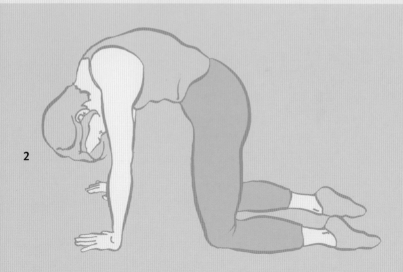

㉒ Glute stretches

Stretches the buttocks, hips and waist

Caution: If you suffer from a knee complaint, take care when practising this exercise.

To begin, sit on the mat with your legs crossed in front of you.

1 Relax your knees down, allowing your hips to open. Place your hands on the mat in front of you to stabilize the upper body. Inhale deeply.

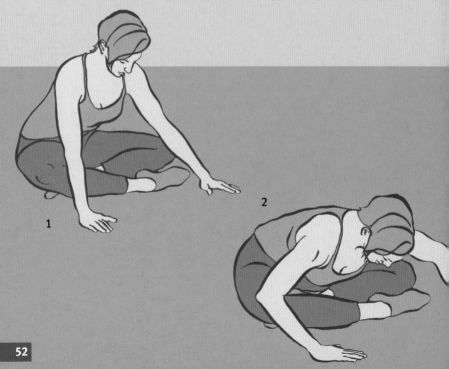

2 As you exhale, lean forwards from the hips, bending the elbows to allow you to stretch further. Hold this position for five deep breaths, gently drawing in the abdominals for extra support.

3 Now twist and stretch the upper body towards the left knee, keeping the right buttock flat on the mat. Hold this position for five deep breaths, again drawing in the abdominals for support. Repeat on the opposite side, crossing the legs the other way.

• **ADVANCED** For a more powerful stretch, adjust the position of the left leg so that the ankle rests on top of the right knee (*see below*).

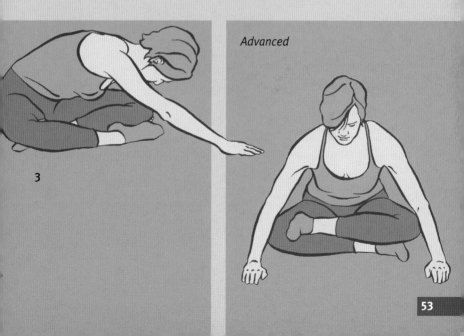

Advanced

3

㉓ Hip stretches

Stretches the hip flexors and the fronts of the thighs

Begin by kneeling on the mat.

1 Bring the left leg up so that the foot stands just in front of the knee and the right leg is bent behind you. Place both hands on the left knee for support. Inhale. Exhale and push the hips forwards as you lift the chest up, drawing your abdominal muscles back towards your spine to create a deeper stretch. Relax into this stretch for five deep breaths.

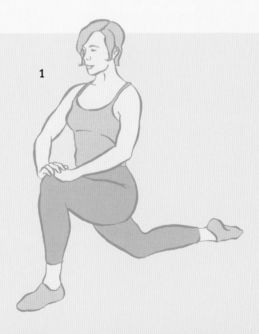

1

2 Raise the right arm and reach over towards the left leg, lifting out of the waist, and stretch the left arm down towards the floor across the inside of the left knee. Exhale, stretching the arms in opposite directions, and take five slow, deep breaths, squeezing the abdominals each time you breathe out.

Repeat to the other side.

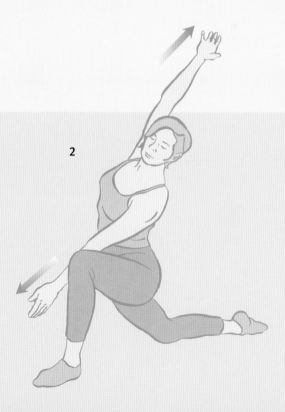

24 Standing side stretches

Stretches the sides of the waist

Stand tall with your feet hip-width apart.

1 Stretch the left arm up towards the ceiling and the right arm down towards the floor. Inhale.

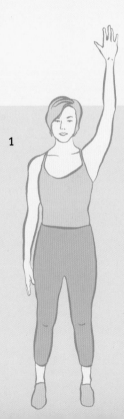

2 As you exhale, reach the left arm over to the right. Focus on the oppositional stretch from the left foot to the left hand. Engage the abdominals to increase the stretch. Release and repeat five times.

3 Repeat five times with the right arm.

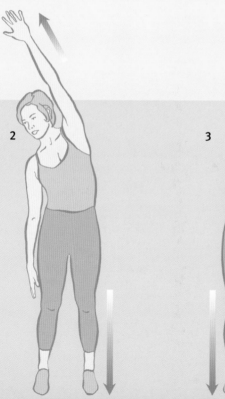

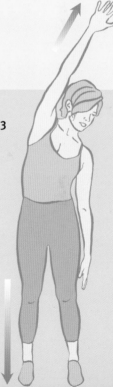

wake up and go

20-MINUTE SESSION

All the exercises in the following routine can be found in the full-length sequence, which you should now be familiar with. The techniques I have selected here will give you boundless energy and leave you feeling ready to face your day!

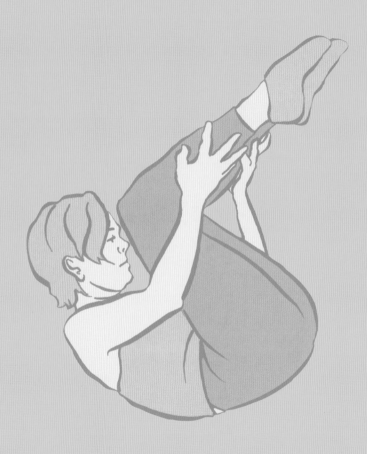

① Breathwork

Helps activate deep postural muscles • Focuses on body alignment and neutral spine

Lie on your back with your knees bent, feet hip-width apart and arms relaxed by your sides. Keeping the shoulders relaxed, gently lengthen the back of your neck and your tailbone, sinking them into the mat so that your spine is resting in neutral. You can find your neutral spine position by slipping one hand under your lower back, into the small space between your body and the floor. Don't over-arch the back.

1 Slowly inhale through your nose, drawing the air deep into your lungs and into the sides of the ribcage – think low and wide.

1

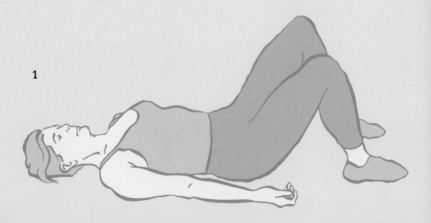

2 Exhale through your mouth and simultaneously pull up through your pelvic floor while squeezing the abdominals down towards your spine as if you are tightening a belt around your waist – try to draw the front of your ribs together at the end of the exhale. Think 'navel to spine' without rocking the pelvis or hunching the shoulders.

Repeat ten times.

Throughout this exercise the breath should not be forced. Create ease and flow, even while engaging the core muscles.

• This breathing technique will be incorporated into the exercise sequences that follow.

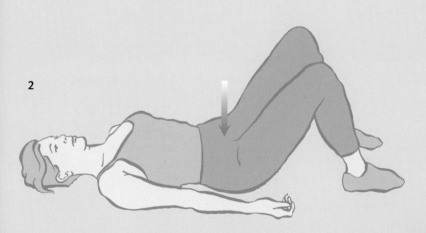

2

❷ The pelvic rock

Mobilizes the pelvis and lower spine • Coordinates breathwork with movement

The pelvic rock is very similar to the breathwork exercise shown on the previous page, but here the pelvis rocks forwards and backwards slightly.

Lie on your back with your knees bent, feet hip-width apart and arms relaxed by your sides. Relax your shoulders and spine into the neutral position by gently lengthening the back of your neck and your tailbone, sinking them into the mat.

1 Inhale deeply, drawing the breath into the sides of the ribcage.

1

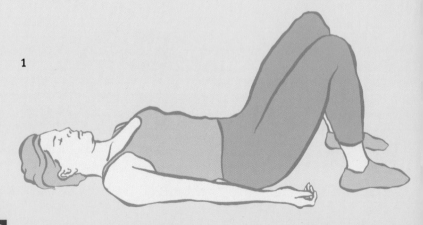

2 As you exhale, draw up through your pelvic floor, engage your abdominals (not your buttocks or hip flexors), lowering them towards the spine, and tilt the pelvis towards the navel slowly rolling the tailbone off the floor. Inhale and release the tailbone back to the neutral position, taking care not to over-exaggerate the curve in the lower spine.

Repeat step 2 ten times.

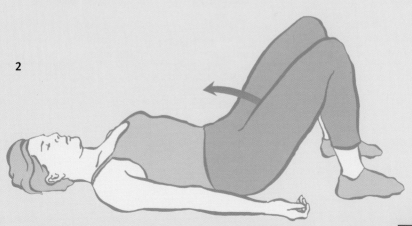

2

❸ The pelvic tilt

Mobilizes and lengthens all the muscles in the spine • Focuses on deep abdominal connection

This is a continuation of the pelvic rock, but now utilizing the whole spine.

Lie on your back in the neutral position with your knees bent, feet hip-width apart and arms relaxed by your sides.

1 Inhale deeply, drawing the breath into the sides of the ribcage.

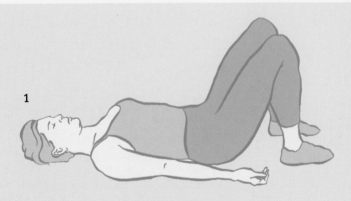

1

2 With a long, sustained exhale, engage your pelvic floor and abdominals and tilt the pelvis towards the navel – the abdominals initiate this movement, not the buttocks. Slowly peel your back off the mat, rolling up through one vertebra at a time. Take care not to lift your pelvis too high as this will cause the back to over-arch. Keep your shoulders and neck relaxed.

3 Inhale, holding this position. Then, as you slowly exhale, roll down one vertebra at a time, lowering the back to the floor, stretching and lengthening through the spine.

Repeat ten times.

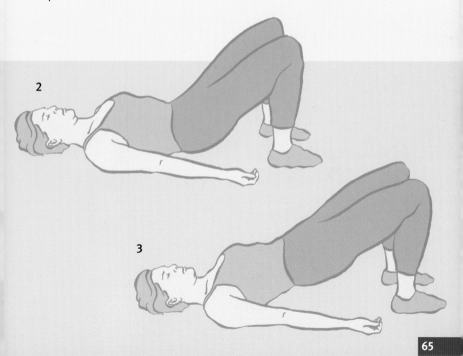

④ Arm reaches

Mobilizes and stabilizes the shoulder blades • Stretches the muscles in the upper and mid back

Lie on your back in the neutral position with your knees bent, feet hip-width apart. Lengthen the back of the neck by drawing the shoulders down away from the ears. The shoulder blades should feel wide apart and flat against the mat. This is your fixed neutral shoulder position.

1 Inhale and stretch the arms up towards the ceiling, pulling the shoulder blades apart to open the upper back. Take care not to hunch the shoulders up towards the ears.

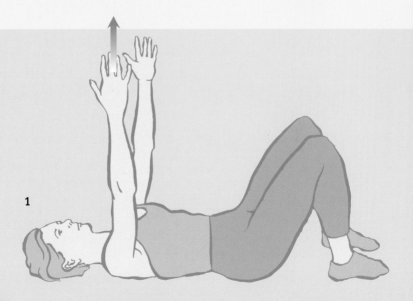

1

2 As you exhale, drop the shoulder blades back to the neutral starting position. Make sure you don't arch the back in response to these subtle movements.

Repeat ten times, concentrating on maintaining the width across the upper back and chest.

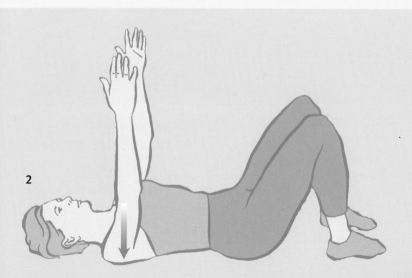

2

⑤ Around the world

Mobilizes the shoulder joints • Opens up the chest and mid back

Caution: Avoid this exercise if you have a history of shoulder dislocation.

For this exercise you may wish to place a small folded towel under your head to keep your neck aligned with the upper back.

1   Lie on your right-hand side with your knees bent, legs together and your arms stretched out in front of you with your palms together.

2   Keeping your knees together, in a slow fluid motion begin to circle the left arm around towards your head. The eyes should follow the arm, but keep your head relaxed and resting on the towel.

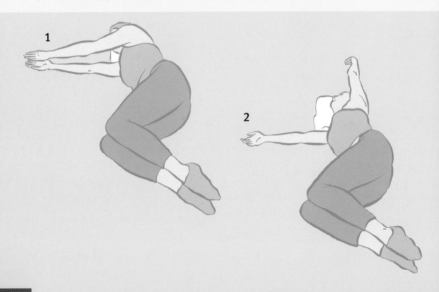

3 Continue to move the arm around, flattening both shoulder blades against the mat as you reach the floor behind you. You should feel a wonderful stretch in the mid back as you gently twist the spine.

4 Finally, bring the arm around past the upper hip and back to the starting position.

Repeat ten times, then complete ten rotations in the opposite direction. Turn over and repeat on the other side.

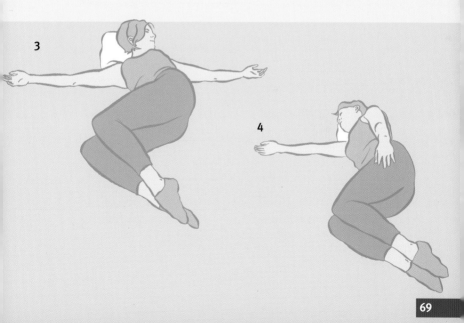

❻ Hundreds

Promotes breath control • Strengthens abdominal and postural muscles • Stabilizes shoulders and pelvis

To help release tension in your neck, place a small folded towel underneath your head before you start. Lie on your back in the neutral position with your knees bent, feet hip-width apart.

1 Place your arms by your sides, slightly raised off the mat, palms facing downwards. Start pumping your arms up and down in a continuous movement, as though you're slapping a puddle on the floor. Focus on keeping your breathing constant.

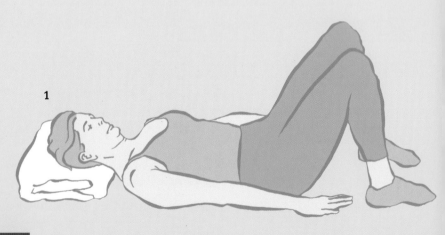

1

2 Inhale deeply for a count of five, then exhale for a count of five, pulling up through your pelvic floor and squeezing your abdominals. Keep your arms strong and stretch your fingers towards your feet. Don't allow the neck to become tense. Each time you exhale, feel all the air being squeezed out of your lungs.

Continue for ten inhales and exhales.

2

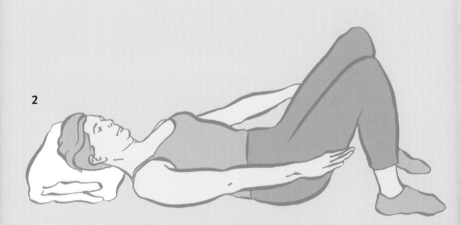

⑦ Rolling like a ball

Maintains abdominal connection while mobilizing the spine

Begin by sitting on the floor at the front of your mat.

1 Draw the knees up towards the chest with your toes resting on the mat. Your body weight should be on your tailbone slightly. Try to create a deep scoop with your abdominals. Place your hands on the outside of the calf muscles.

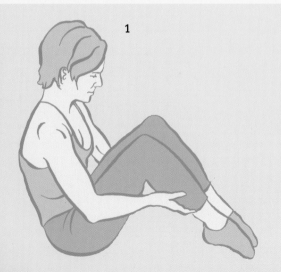

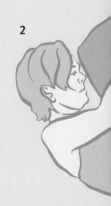

2 Maintaining this scooped position with your chin pointed down towards your chest, inhale and begin to roll back onto your shoulder blades – don't allow your head to touch the mat.

3 Immediately roll back up to the position shown in step 1. As you roll up, exhale using your abdominal muscles. You will find it easier to roll through your spine if you keep your heels close to your buttocks and your chin towards your chest.

Repeat ten times.

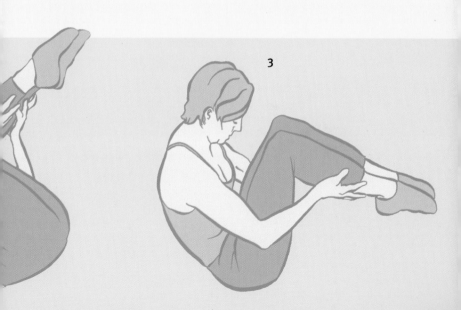

3

⑧ The spine stretch

Mobilizes and lengthens the spine • Stretches the hamstrings

Begin by sitting with your legs slightly wider than hip-width apart, knees slightly bent.

1 Reach your arms out in front of you, level with your shoulders. Focus on lengthening your spine upwards and draw your shoulders down towards the hips. If you find this difficult, bend your knees a little more, keeping your feet flat on the floor. Inhale deeply into the ribcage.

2 As you exhale, squeeze the abdominals back towards the spine and curve your whole spine forwards, reaching the hands towards the toes

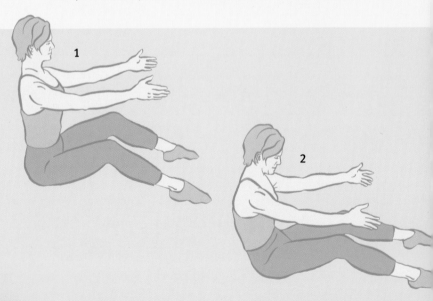

– imagine that your waist is being pulled back as you stretch forwards. Try not to hunch the shoulders – keep them away from the ears.

3 Inhale, keeping the abdominal muscles scooped in, and focus on maximizing the stretch.

4 Exhale and roll the spine back up, one vertebra at a time, to return to the upright position shown in step 1.

Repeat ten times.

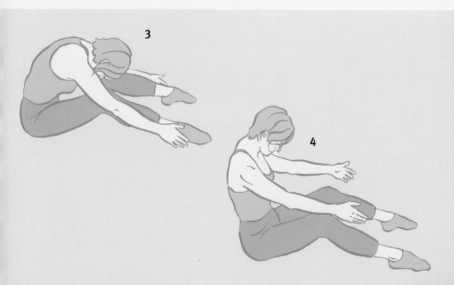

⑨ The cat

Mobilizes and stretches the spine • Stabilizes the shoulders

On all fours, position your hands directly underneath the shoulders and place your knees in line with the hips.

1   Look down towards the floor so that your head is in line with the neck and draw the shoulders away from the ears. Lengthen your spine in both directions. Inhale deeply into the ribcage.

1

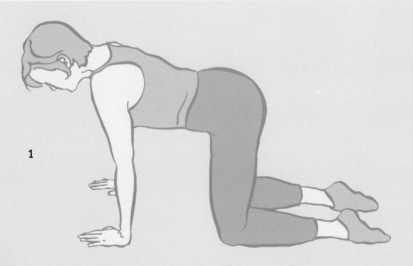

2 Exhale, pulling up through your pelvic floor, and squeeze your abdominals back towards your spine lifting the spine up towards the ceiling. At the top of this lift, inhale, gently pressing the hands down into the mat to achieve a greater stretch. Exhale and relax the spine down to the starting position.

Repeat ten times.

2

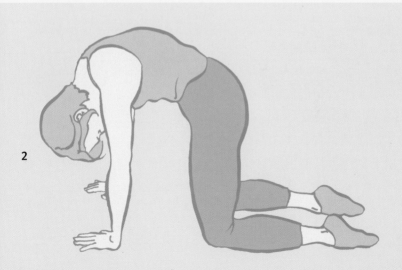

⑩ Glute stretches

Stretches the buttocks, hips and waist

Caution: If you suffer from a knee complaint, take care when practising this exercise.

To begin, sit on the mat with your legs crossed in front of you.

1 Relax your knees down, allowing your hips to open. Place your hands on the mat in front of you to stabilize the upper body. Inhale deeply.

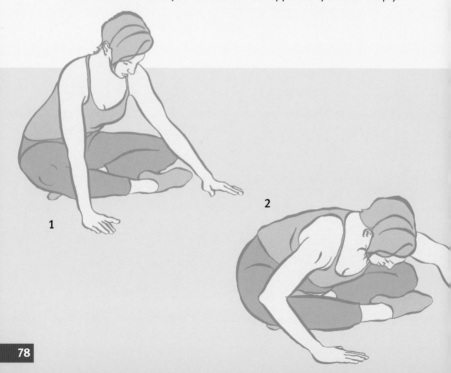

1

2

2   As you exhale, lean forwards from the hips, bending the elbows to allow you to stretch further. Hold this position for five deep breaths, gently drawing in the abdominals for extra support.

3   Now twist and stretch the upper body towards the left knee, keeping the right buttock flat on the mat. Hold this position for five deep breaths, again drawing in the abdominals for support. Repeat on the opposite side, crossing the legs the other way.

ADVANCED   For a more powerful stretch, adjust the position of the left leg so that the ankle rests on top of the right knee (*see below*).

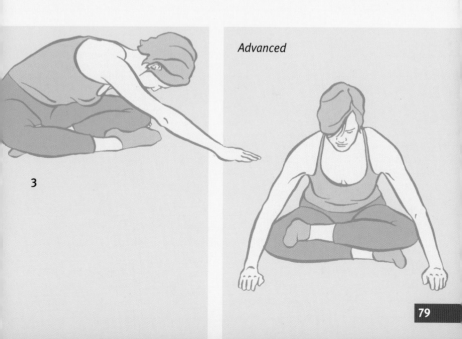

Advanced

3

⑪ Hip stretches

Stretches the hip flexors and the fronts of the thighs

Begin by kneeling on the mat.

1 Bring the left leg up so that the foot stands just in front of the knee and the right leg is bent behind you. Place both hands on the left knee for support. Inhale. Exhale and push the hips forwards as you lift the chest up, drawing your abdominal muscles back towards your spine to create a deeper stretch. Relax into this stretch for five deep breaths.

1

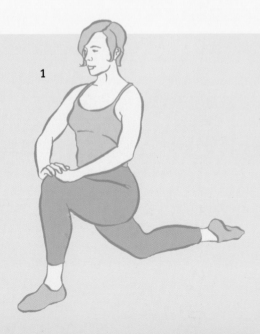

2 Raise the right arm and reach over towards the left leg, lifting out of the waist, and stretch the left arm down towards the floor across the inside of the left knee. Exhale, stretching the arms in opposite directions, and take five slow, deep breaths, squeezing the abdominals each time you breathe out.

Repeat to the other side.

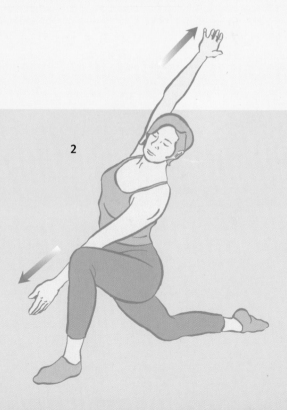

2

⑫ Standing side stretches

Stretches the sides of the waist

Stand tall with your feet hip-width apart.

1 Stretch the left arm up towards the ceiling and the right arm down towards the floor. Inhale.

1

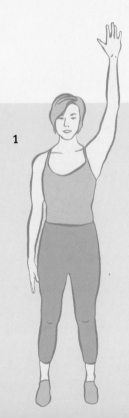

2 As you exhale, reach the left arm over to the right. Focus on the oppositional stretch from the left foot to the left hand. Engage the abdominals to increase the stretch. Release and repeat five times.

3 Repeat five times with the right arm.

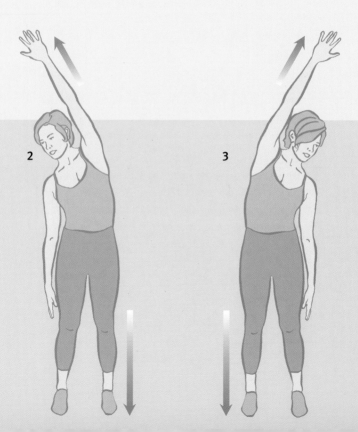

shoulders and neck

10-MINUTE SESSION

This routine includes some exercises which can be found in the full-length sequence, as well as some new ones that are particularly beneficial to the shoulders and neck. The new exercises are indicated by a ❖ at the top of the page.

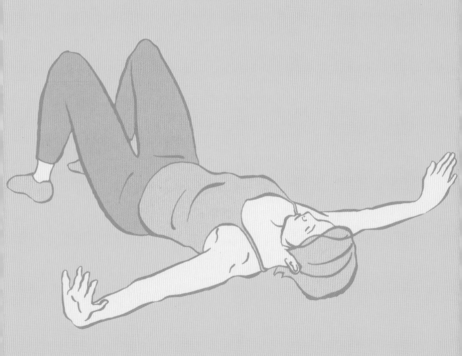

❶ Breathwork

Helps activate deep postural muscles • Focuses on body alignment and neutral spine

Lie on your back with your knees bent, feet hip-width apart and arms relaxed by your sides. Keeping the shoulders relaxed, gently lengthen the back of your neck and your tailbone, sinking them into the mat so that your spine is resting in neutral. You can find your neutral spine position by slipping one hand under your lower back, into the small space between your body and the floor. Don't over-arch the back.

1   Slowly inhale through your nose, drawing the air deep into your lungs and into the sides of the ribcage – think low and wide.

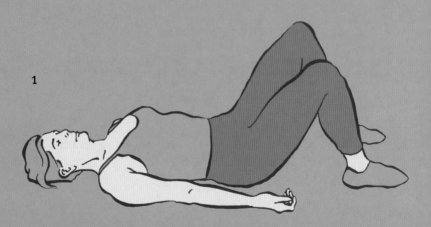

1

2 Exhale through your mouth and simultaneously pull up through your pelvic floor while squeezing the abdominals down towards your spine as if you are tightening a belt around your waist – try to draw the front of your ribs together at the end of the exhale. Think 'navel to spine' without rocking the pelvis or hunching the shoulders.

Repeat ten times.

Throughout this exercise the breath should not be forced. Create ease and flow, even while engaging the core muscles.

- This breathing technique will be incorporated into the exercise sequences that follow.

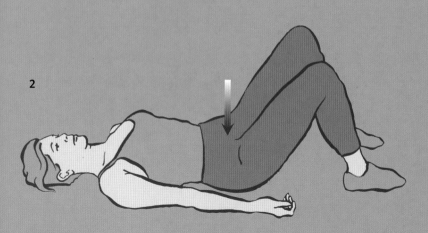

2

❷ Chin nods

Helps stretch and lengthen the back of the neck • Releases tension in the neck and shoulders

Lie on your back with your knees bent and your feet hip-width apart. Your arms should be by your sides.

1 Relax your spine in the neutral position, releasing any tension in the fronts of the hips. Stretch your arms towards your feet. Inhale, dropping the shoulders away from the ears to lengthen the back of the neck.

1

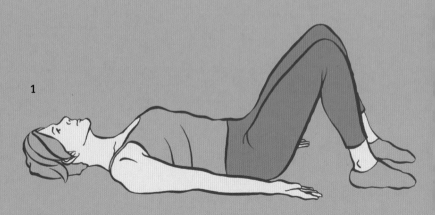

2 As you exhale, lower the chin towards the chest and gently stretch the back of the neck towards the mat. Take care not to arch your back. Inhale and release the chin back to the neutral position. To gain maximum benefit from this subtle exercise, keep the shoulders relaxed throughout.

Repeat ten times.

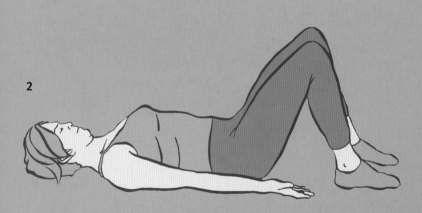

2

❸ Arm reaches

Mobilizes and stabilizes the shoulder blades • Stretches the muscles in the upper and mid back

Lie on your back in the neutral position with your knees bent, feet hip-width apart. Lengthen the back of the neck by drawing the shoulders down away from the ears. The shoulder blades should feel wide apart and flat against the mat. This is your fixed neutral shoulder position.

1 Inhale and stretch the arms up towards the ceiling, pulling the shoulder blades apart to open the upper back. Take care not to hunch the shoulders up towards the ears.

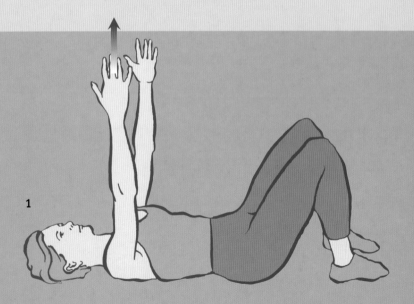

2 As you exhale, drop the shoulder blades back to the neutral starting position. Make sure you don't arch the back in response to these subtle movements.

Repeat ten times, concentrating on maintaining the width across the upper back and chest.

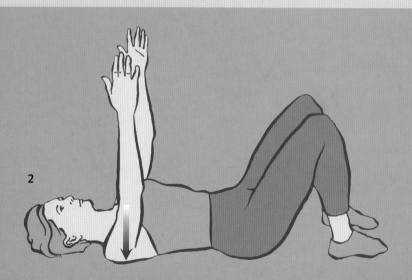

❹ Nerve stretches

Releases tension in the neck and shoulders

Lie on your back with your knees bent and your feet hip-width apart.

1 Reach your arms out to the sides, level with your shoulders, palms facing down. Relax your spine in the neutral position, releasing any tension in the front of the hips. Inhale and lengthen the back of your neck, sliding the shoulders away from your ears.

1

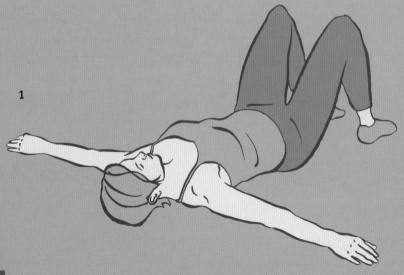

2 As you exhale, bend the wrists to lift the palms off the mat and extend the fingers up towards the ceiling as if you are pushing against a door frame. Feel the energy being pushing out through your palms. Try not to arch the back and keep your arms and wrists on the mat. Inhale to release.

Repeat ten times.

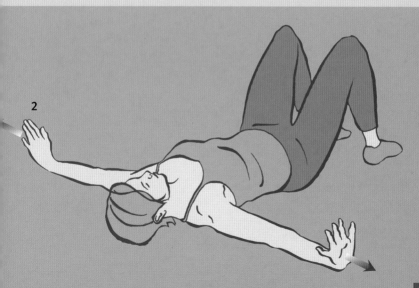

2

❺ Around the world

Mobilizes the shoulder joints • Opens up the chest and mid back

Caution: Avoid this exercise if you have a history of shoulder dislocation.

For this exercise you may wish to place a small folded towel under your head to keep your neck aligned with the upper back.

1 Lie on your right-hand side with your knees bent, legs together and your arms stretched out in front of you with your palms together.

2 Keeping your knees together, in a slow fluid motion begin to circle the left arm around towards your head. The eyes should follow the arm, but keep your head relaxed and resting on the towel.

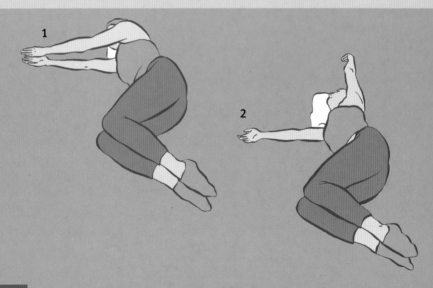

3 Continue to move the arm around, flattening both shoulder blades against the mat as you reach the floor behind you. You should feel a wonderful stretch in the mid back as you gently twist the spine.

4 Finally, bring the arm around past the upper hip and back to the starting position.

Repeat ten times, then complete ten rotations in the opposite direction. Turn over and repeat on the other side.

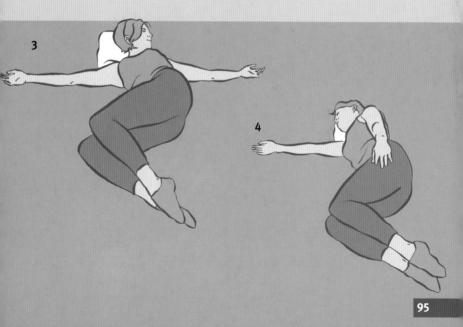

❻ Single-arm lifts

Strengthens core postural muscles • Stabilizes the shoulder blades

Begin by getting on all fours, placing your hands directly underneath your shoulders and your knees in line with your hips.

1 Look down towards the floor so that your head is in line with your neck, and draw your shoulders away from the ears. Lengthen your spine in both directions – out through the crown of your head and the tailbone. Inhale deeply into the ribcage.

1

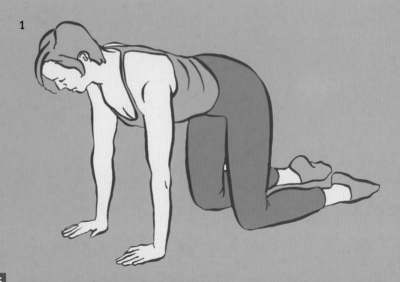

2 As you exhale, pull up through your pelvic floor and squeeze your abdominals back towards your spine. Now lift the left hand off the floor and press both shoulders down towards your hips. Keep the spine in a neutral position. This is essential to gain maximum benefit from the exercise. Focus on maintaining your core centre so that your weight doesn't shift to one side. Inhale and place your hand back on the mat.

Repeat ten times, alternating sides.

2

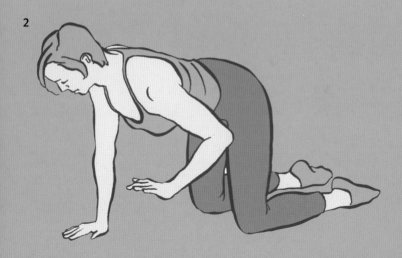

❼ The cat

Mobilizes and stretches the spine • Stabilizes the shoulders

On all fours, position your hands directly underneath the shoulders and place your knees in line with the hips.

1 Look down towards the floor so that your head is in line with the neck and draw the shoulders away from the ears. Lengthen your spine in both directions. Inhale deeply into the ribcage.

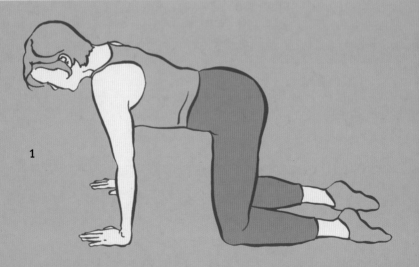

1

2 Exhale, pulling up through your pelvic floor, and squeeze your
  abdominals back towards your spine lifting the spine up towards the
  ceiling. At the top of this lift, inhale, gently pressing the hands down
  into the mat to achieve a greater stretch. Exhale and relax the spine
  down to the starting position.

Repeat ten times.

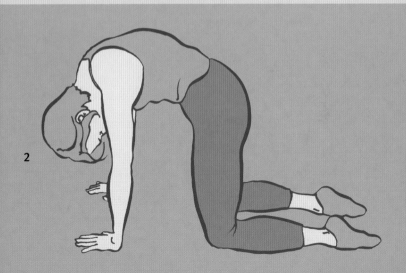

2

❽ The cobra

*Strengthens the core abdominal and back muscles • Stabilizes
the shoulder blades*

Begin by lying face down with your legs hip-width apart.

1 Place your palms face down next to your shoulders and rest your elbows
   by your sides, close to the ribs. Gently press the elbows down into the
   mat. Slide the shoulder blades downwards and outwards towards your
   hips, fixing the shoulders away from the ears. Look down to lengthen
   the back of the neck, and stretch the spine in both directions. Inhale,
   focusing on this spinal stretch.

1

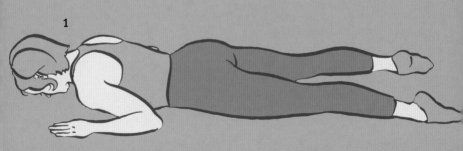

2 As you exhale, pull up through your pelvic floor and squeeze your navel towards the spine. Lift the chest off the mat and keep your elbows pressed down. It is imperative to maintain the connection in the abdominals at this point to ensure sufficient support for the lower back. Inhale and lower the body back down to the mat.

Repeat ten times.

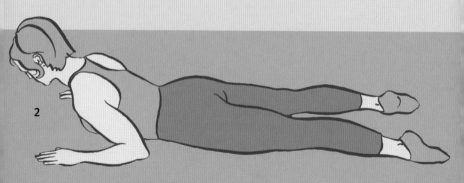

2

❾ Threading the needle

Stretches the upper and mid back

Begin on all fours, positioning your hands directly underneath your shoulders, with the fingers pointing towards each other. Look down towards the floor so that your head is in line with your neck and draw your shoulders away from your ears.

1 Inhale, turning the right palm up towards the ceiling.

2 As you exhale, slide the back of the hand along the mat and through the gap behind the stabilizing arm.

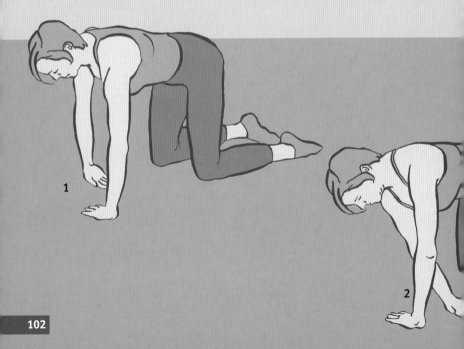

3 Stretch the right arm through until the back of the shoulder is as close to the floor as possible. Bend the elbow of the stabilizing arm to create more stretch and length in the right shoulder. Try to keep the hips directly over the knees while rotating the spine. Inhale, increasing the stretch through the finger tips, then exhale to return to the starting position.

Repeat ten times, alternating sides.

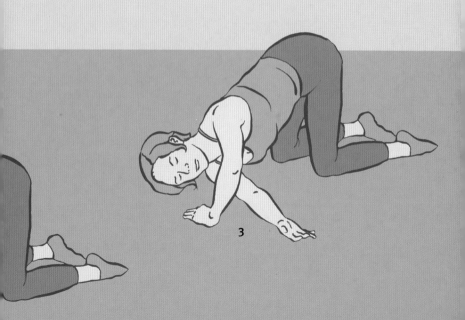

3

⑩ The drinking lion

Stretches the upper and mid back and shoulders

Begin by getting on all fours, propping yourself up on your elbows.

1 Press your hands together in the prayer position. Inhale.

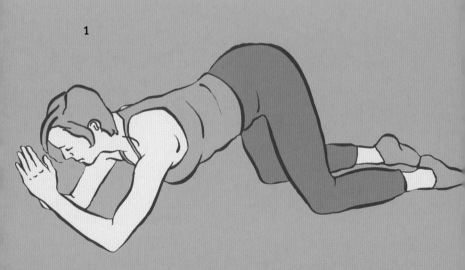

1

2 As you exhale, drop your chest and chin down towards the floor while reaching your finger tips and hips up towards the ceiling – don't allow your hips to fall back towards your heels. Relax into the stretch for a few seconds. Inhale to return to the starting position.

Repeat five times.

2

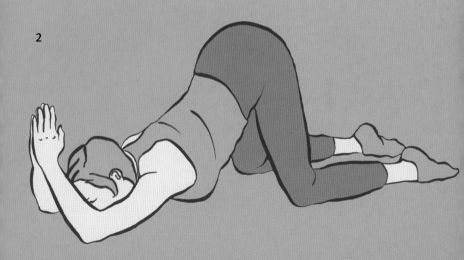

lower back

10-MINUTE SESSION

The majority of the exercises included in this routine are found in the full-length sequence. There is just one new exercise – the single-leg slides – which is particularly beneficial to the lower back.

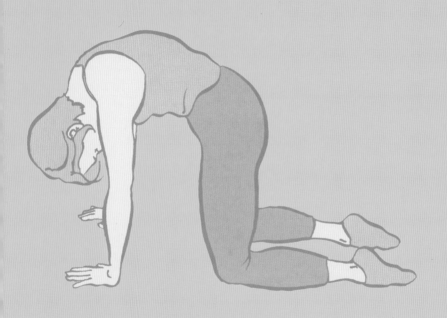

① Breathwork

Helps activate deep postural muscles • Focuses on body alignment and neutral spine

Lie on your back with your knees bent, feet hip-width apart and arms relaxed by your sides. Keeping the shoulders relaxed, gently lengthen the back of your neck and your tailbone, sinking them into the mat so that your spine is resting in neutral. You can find your neutral spine position by slipping one hand under your lower back, into the small space between your body and the floor. Don't over-arch the back.

1 Slowly inhale through your nose, drawing the air deep into your lungs and into the sides of the ribcage – think low and wide.

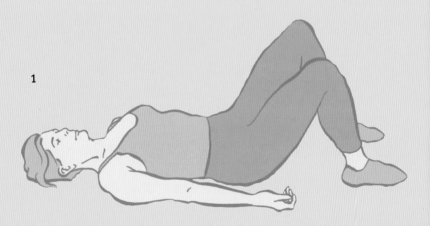

1

2 Exhale through your mouth and simultaneously pull up through your pelvic floor while squeezing the abdominals down towards your spine as if you are tightening a belt around your waist – try to draw the front of your ribs together at the end of the exhale. Think 'navel to spine' without rocking the pelvis or hunching the shoulders.

Repeat ten times.

Throughout this exercise the breath should not be forced. Create ease and flow, even while engaging the core muscles.

• This breathing technique will be incorporated into the exercise sequences that follow.

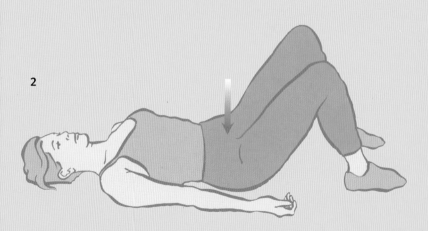

2

❷ The pelvic rock

Mobilizes the pelvis and lower spine • Coordinates breathwork with movement

The pelvic rock is very similar to the breathwork exercise shown on the previous page, but here the pelvis rocks forwards and backwards slightly.

Lie on your back with your knees bent, feet hip-width apart and arms relaxed by your sides. Relax your shoulders and spine into the neutral position by gently lengthening the back of your neck and your tailbone, sinking them into the mat.

1 Inhale deeply, drawing the breath into the sides of the ribcage.

1

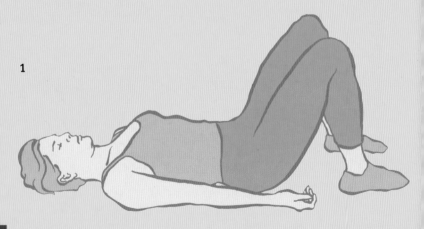

2 As you exhale, draw up through your pelvic floor, engage your abdominals (not your buttocks or hip flexors), lowering them towards the spine, and tilt the pelvis towards the navel slowly rolling the tailbone off the floor. Inhale and release the tailbone back to the neutral position, taking care not to over-exaggerate the curve in the lower spine.

Repeat step 2 ten times.

2

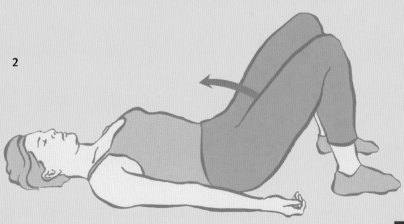

❸ Knee drops

Stabilizes the pelvis • Mobilizes the hip joints

This exercise requires you to stabilize one side of your body, while mobilizing the other.

1 Lie on your back in the neutral position with your knees bent, feet hip-width apart and arms relaxed by your sides. Focus on the pelvic floor and abdominal muscles to maintain a neutral pelvis throughout. Keep your neck relaxed.

2 As you inhale, relax one knee out to the side, making sure the opposite hip doesn't lift from the floor.

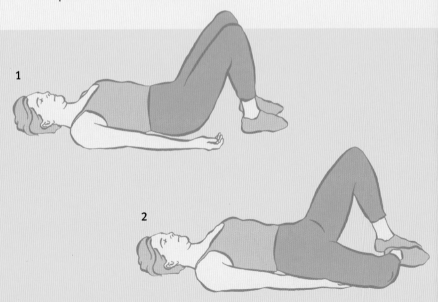

3 Exhale and extend the leg along the mat, taking care not to arch the back – think of the stretch starting from the hip. Keep the leg extended as you inhale.

4 As you exhale, pull the navel down towards the spine, and, primarily using the abdominal muscles, bend the leg back to the starting position keeping the foot on the mat.

Repeat ten times with each leg.

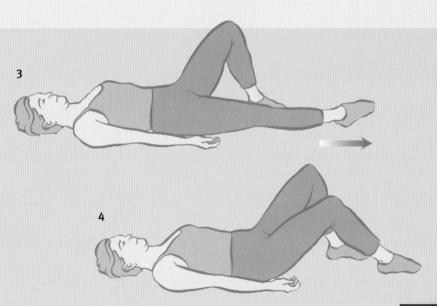

❹ Single-leg slides

Stretches out the sides and the backs of the hips

Begin by lying on your right-hand side.

1 Straighten out your left leg and bend your right knee so that your upper leg is level with the hip. Stretch out your right arm as shown below and rest your head on the arm. Place your left hand on the mat in front of your chest. Inhale.

1

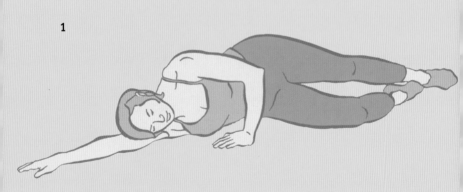

2 As you exhale, stretch your left leg downwards away from your shoulder, sliding the leg along the mat. Keep the leg straight and the foot on the mat. The left hip will stretch down with the movement of the leg, releasing the muscles in the surrounding area. Inhale to gently glide the hip back to the starting position.

Repeat ten times, then complete the whole exercise on the other side.

2

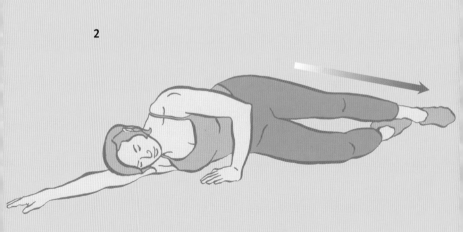

⑤ The cat

Mobilizes and stretches the spine • Stabilizes the shoulders

On all fours, position your hands directly underneath the shoulders and place your knees in line with the hips.

1 Look down towards the floor so that your head is in line with the neck and draw the shoulders away from the ears. Lengthen your spine in both directions. Inhale deeply into the ribcage.

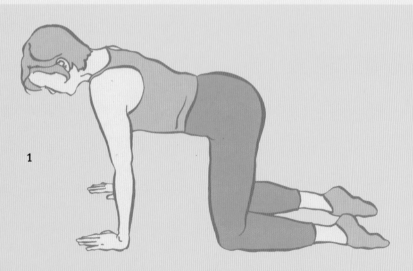

1

2 Exhale, pulling up through your pelvic floor, and squeeze your abdominals back towards your spine lifting the spine up towards the ceiling. At the top of this lift, inhale, gently pressing the hands down into the mat to achieve a greater stretch. Exhale and relax the spine down to the starting position.

Repeat ten times.

2

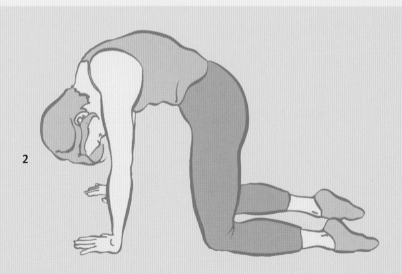

⑥ Superman

Stabilizes the shoulder blades • Strengthens the core abdominal and back muscles • Works the hamstrings and buttocks

On all fours, position your hands directly underneath your shoulders and place your knees in line with your hips.

1 Look down towards the floor so that your head is in line with the neck and draw the shoulders away from the ears. Lengthen your spine in both directions. Inhale deeply into the ribcage.

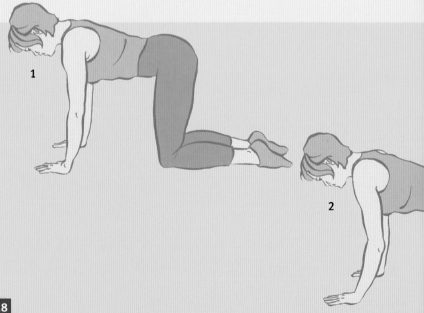

2 As you exhale, pull up through your pelvic floor and squeeze your abdominals back towards your spine. Then lift your right leg off the floor, extending it straight back in line with the hip. Try not to shift your weight to the left or lift the right hip – it's important to maintain the neutral pelvis. Inhale, holding this position.

3 Exhale and raise the left hand. Once again, concentrate on keeping your weight centred and your shoulders pressed down, away from your ears. As you inhale, return your arm and leg to the starting position shown in step 1.

Repeat ten times alternating sides.

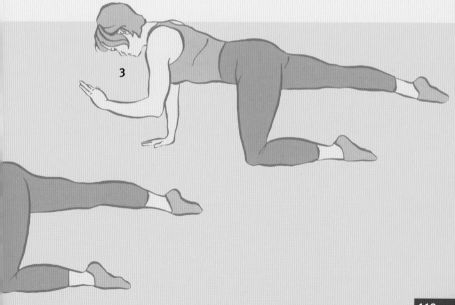

⑦ The star

Strengthens the core muscle groups • Lengthens the spine • Works the hamstrings and buttocks

Begin by lying face down on the mat.

1   Place your legs hip-width apart and extend your arms out in front of you, shoulder-width apart, palms flat on the mat. Look down to lengthen the back of the neck and pull your shoulders down away from the ears. Inhale, fixing the shoulder blades down towards the hips.

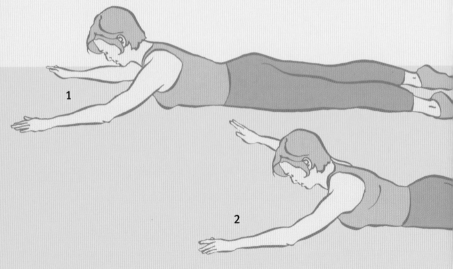

2 As you exhale, pull up through the pelvic floor and squeeze the navel back towards the spine. This will ensure that the lower back is adequately supported. Simultaneously, lift and lengthen the right arm and left leg. Make sure both hips remain on the mat. Inhale and lower the arm and leg back down to the mat.

3 Repeat step 2 with the left arm and right leg.

Repeat five times.

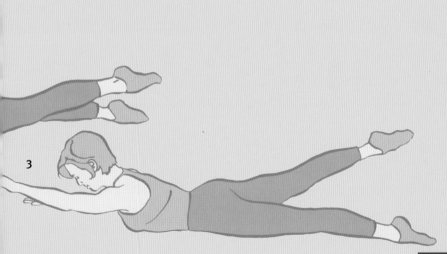

8 Glute stretches

Stretches the buttocks, hips and waist

Caution: If you suffer from a knee complaint, take care when practising this exercise.

To begin, sit on the mat with your legs crossed in front of you.

1 Relax your knees down, allowing your hips to open. Place your hands on the mat in front of you to stabilize the upper body. Inhale deeply.

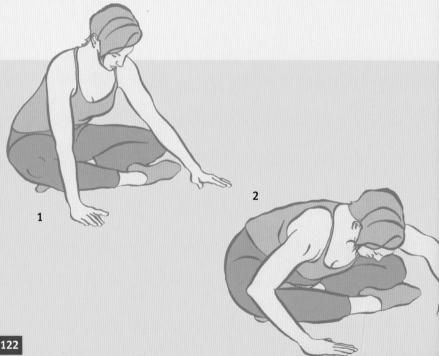

2 As you exhale, lean forwards from the hips, bending the elbows to allow you to stretch further. Hold this position for five deep breaths, gently drawing in the abdominals for extra support.

3 Now twist and stretch the upper body towards the left knee, keeping the right buttock flat on the mat. Hold this position for five deep breaths, again drawing in the abdominals for support. Repeat on the opposite side, crossing the legs the other way.

ADVANCED For a more powerful stretch, adjust the position of the left leg so that the ankle rests on top of the right knee (*see below*).

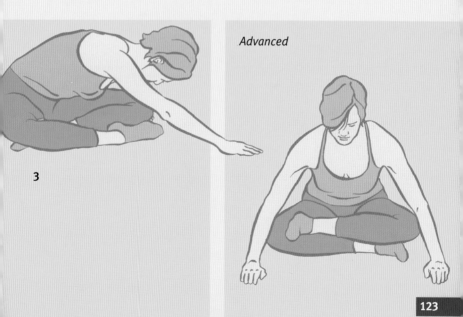

Advanced

3

⑨ Hip stretches

Stretches the hip flexors and the fronts of the thighs

Begin by kneeling on the mat.

1 Bring the left leg up so that the foot stands just in front of the knee and the right leg is bent behind you. Place both hands on the left knee for support. Inhale. Exhale and push the hips forwards as you lift the chest up, drawing your abdominal muscles back towards your spine to create a deeper stretch. Relax into this stretch for five deep breaths.

1

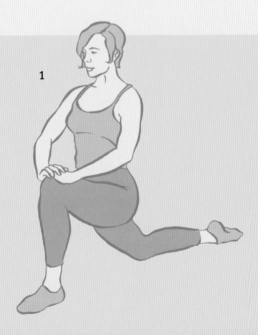

2 Raise the right arm and reach over towards the left leg, lifting out of the waist, and stretch the left arm down towards the floor across the inside of the left knee. Exhale, stretching the arms in opposite directions, and take five slow, deep breaths, squeezing the abdominals each time you breathe out.

Repeat to the other side.

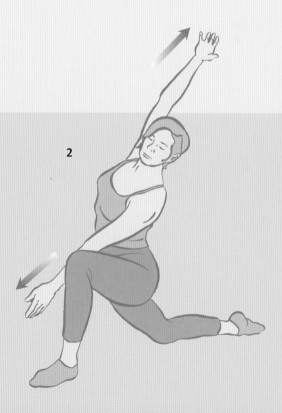

⑩ Standing side stretches

Stretches the sides of the waist

Stand tall with your feet hip-width apart.

1 Stretch the left arm up towards the ceiling and the right arm down
   towards the floor. Inhale.

1

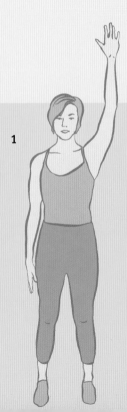

2 As you exhale, reach the left arm over to the right. Focus on the oppositional stretch from the left foot to the left hand. Engage the abdominals to increase the stretch. Release and repeat five times.

3 Repeat five times with the right arm.

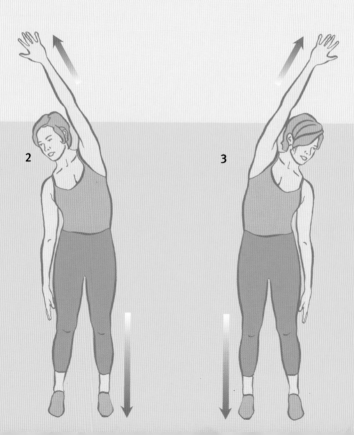

ABOUT THE AUTHOR

Mina Stephens has more than 20 years' Pilates experience. While working as a professional dancer in New York, she trained with renowned master Pilates teachers, Romana Kryzanowska and Sean P. Gallagher. Her dance career took her to Paris and she eventually set down roots in London. Mina received her Pilates teaching diploma with Dominique Jansen at Pilates off the Square, a studio accredited with the Pilates Foundation. Mina now has her own studio in Notting Hill, Pilates @ Float, where she mainly works with private clients. She is also a Reiki healer – this and her extensive worldwide training have helped her to develop a unique holistic and rehabilitative approach to her teaching.

ABOUT THE CONSULTANT

Sean Durkan has a BSc degree from the London School of Osteopathy, and is a member of the General Osteopathic Council. He has been in practice for seven years at Harley Street, London, and he also has residency at the Queen's Tennis Club, London, where he treats sports professionals; his clients also include many actors and musicians. Sean takes a holistic approach to osteopathy, looking at clients' posture, dietary habits and general lifestyle as a way to improve well-being. His personal interests include Pilates and yoga.

ACKNOWLEDGEMENTS

Many thanks to Katie Golsby and Malcolm Smythe for their patience and advice, and to Sean Durkan for his professional input. And lastly, thanks to my parents for their incredible love and support.